Table of Contents

The Impact of Rain on Allergies

1. Introduction to Allergies and Rain

Rain often has either a positive or negative effect on allergies. People can experience either relief or a surge in asthma and allergy symptoms when the air composition changes due to the interaction of rain and plants. The total amount of pollen grains in the air lowers due to the increased humidity during rain. However, many plants release or put the pollen grains in the air before the rain starts falling - during the 'clean-up time' - right after an increase in temperature and shrink end. Besides, a sudden drop in humidity - especially during thunderstorms - releases the pollen grains into the air. This surge in asthma and allergies can translate into a constant cough, wheezing, itchy and runny nose, teary or itchy eyes, a sore throat, a headache, tiredness, and an asthma attack that can lead to a hospital visit. The rain can do this by breaking pollen grains into tiny particles inside the humid air, acting as bullets to the immune system for unfortunate allergic people, or when sucking the pollen grains up to the clouds and returning them in the form of raindrops loaded with pollen to the ground. Moreover, molds can grow in gardens, riverbeds, gutters, and the soil due to the humidity and water of the rain. Mold releases spores into the air that can also be inhaled and induce asthma and allergies.

Many people experience an increase in allergy symptoms when it rains. This article digs deeper into the effects that rain has on both outdoor and indoor allergies. There are meals, stress-relief tactics, and preventative measures that can help. This article will focus on the rain's effects on outdoor allergies and deal with indoor allergies in another post.

2. How Rain Can Aggravate Allergies

Heavy rainfall may also drop some of the heavy pollen performer particles to the ground, but unbloomed buds, flowers, and grass can pose a higher threat to allergy sufferers in a humid environment. Low humidity levels show less of this scenario. Mold also becomes a major threat as a result of rainy weather. With the addition of rain, mold spores can become airborne and spread more widely in the atmosphere. The colonies of mold spores trapped on outdoor and indoor surfaces can extend to larger masses of allergies. Lastly, rain can also trigger grasses and flowering plants, such as ragweed, which release small spores into the wind during dry conditions that follow a rainy period, exacerbating allergic sensitivity. In conclusion, humidity can bring relief to some, but it can make it harder for others. In addition, growing plants and greenery may make allergic reactions more severe due to the dryness brought by rainfall.

Rain is often thought of as a cleanser that rids the environment of impurities. However, for many allergy sufferers, it can exacerbate symptoms and leave behind more lingering problems. This happens because when it rains, pollen in the air may remain longer than usual and it becomes prone to bursting and releasing its contents. These small particles of pollen then quickly spread throughout the area and may cause further allergies among people. All the surfaces such as railings, walls, and benches may contain pollen residue as the rain dries out and the wind blows the tiny pollen particles everywhere from your surrounding plants. Lastly, clouds, which are large masses, may shelve and disperse pollen grains just over your heads, thus increasing their lingering effects.

2.1. Washing Pollen Out of the Air

Pollen is not as passive as its lack of color makes it look. If you've ever seen a waterway that suddenly floods and carries all manner of floatables away, you have a clearer idea of what happens when rain hits a tree, dumping a lot of pollen into the air. "A lot of trees are not just releasing pollen throughout the growing season, they're releasing that pollen directly in response to rain," Paul recounts. "Additionally, the amount of pollen that's released is directly correlated to the intensity of the rain," she explains. "If it's a light sprinkle, it's not going to be enough to break up those pollen clumps and blow them around. Instead, it's going to be a hard squall that's chock-full of pollen. And then the other trees will say, 'Thank you very much, that's my cue,' and they'll start releasing their pollen, too."

Rain can exacerbate allergies in a counterintuitive way. "Everybody thinks about hay fever being triggered by the start of the growing season, when plants are in flower," Paul explains. "But in fact, the main factor that triggers my symptoms is the rain." This is apparently not entirely uncommon among polliniferous plants along the East Coast and Southeastern United States. They use rain events to give their windblown pollen an extra boost in spreading, Paul says.

3. Types of Allergens Affected by Rain

Pollen, mold, and fungal spores are all aggravated by damp weather because they require moist conditions for growth. The most common type of allergen impacted by rain is pollen. Most plants naturally release pollen into the air to reproduce, releasing even more if rain is expected soon. Trees typically release pollen in the spring and grasses in the summer, as they need to spread their pollen before growing new leaves or producing seeds. Mold and fungal spores are another type of outdoor allergen that increases in prevalence during and after it rains. Molds thrive in damp conditions and can be found in leaf piles, compost, attics, air vent systems, and anywhere else that has persistent moisture. They release tiny spores into the air that can get into an individual's nose and cause an allergic reaction. Indoor allergens such as dust mites are also more plentiful when it rains. Female dust mites rely on moisture to lay their eggs, and they produce allergens in their fecal matter. When humidity rises, an increase in the growth of mold and bacteria on (and in) their food — bits of shed human skin and pet dander — is also often observed.

When considering how rain affects allergies, an individual might think of rain primarily in its capacity to wash away pollen and other allergens from the air. However, this explanation is simplistic, as many different types of allergens are now known to increase in prevalence after it rains. In recent years, research has shown that many indoor allergens, which are typically less influenced by weather than outdoor allergens, can become more common after rain.

3.1. Pollen

Rain closes with pollen, a major hydrophilic, retaining a fairy that ensures rapid germination and rapid growth of the hini-tube when the pollen grain comes in contact with stigma. The kernels of RNA inherently cause it to agglomerate, buying nupelaț particles and dragging them to the ground. Large particles are deposited on the ground near the conifers, while the small ones can rise after a week and travel away from the mountains. These negatively charged moist particles in the air reduce the concentration of pollen but increase the concentration of ozone and nitrate in the air, leading to smog in urban areas. The pollen kernel can travel long distances because lightning is 20,000 times more charged negative ions, allowing them to obtain matrix mheivia micieux or organic possing tende hat sea. A ken before night, during the rainy can make all pollen and spores are dragged from the air padphillolAxis where a plant may have more than four hundred flowers and release billions of pollen grains.

It's no secret to anyone who suffers from them that springtime is associated with a different kind of cold: allergies. In this section, we discuss allergens, the agents and carriers for these allergies, and their sensitization during the scenario investigations in the background. Allergens are relatively small, mainly proteins that roughly 20% of the world's population cannot tolerate. Dust mites are another food allergen that is particularly common and found in imb of soil (e.g., soil and compost). Molds are particularly serious in baton stokers for allergic ones, scoring as high as mites in the allergens mostly associated with innuse Eitle Houses.

4. Regions Most Affected by Rain-Related Allergies

Your geographic area and the environmental allergens that live there are both contributors to your allergic misery. Regional geography and environmental diversity include dust of hay, tree, grass, weed, and flowers in bloom in the eyes of the allergist. In windy dry weather (a Santa Ana effect), all of the day's allergens are up in the air including dust as a rule. In a mid-April snowstorm of 1986 rife with "gunk", pollen and mold counts like headaches skyrocketed. Better, its horniest example appears in the month. April showers bring May allergies is the adage, rain and all the lousy symptoms that go with the free wash water of the air baths off the trees we'll gratefully keep.

Rain can bring pollen grains to the ground, wash trees of pollen first thing in the morning, and increase the humidity levels that mold spores need to grow. Since rising airborne moisture and scientifically documented pollen counts are a prodrome to rain, those in the know have only to stay indoors on days when an increase in these two intersect under a dark, pendulous rain cloud. Lastly, identical twins' allergies do not act the same on an area-wide basis. Allergen sensitivity and allergic disease are variable from one region to another. Where is the rain and pollen allergy situation worst in the USA? According to the American Academy of Allergy, Asthma, and Immunology, it is always something somewhere. Otherwise, those four physicians see to it when and wherever possible.

5. Strategies to Minimize Allergy Symptoms During Rainy Seasons

Keep pollen away by changing your clothes, washing up, and leaving your shoes at the door. If you have to go outside when the pollen count is high because, for example, you're out of allergy medicine, a mask can help. You should change your home filters no matter what, but if you're avoiding pollen, changing them during allergy season can help. Use a high-efficiency particulate air (HEPA) filter that's specifically designed to reduce pet allergens, pollutants, and pollen. You can put these filters on your air conditioner, your heating system, or your portable air purifier. When it comes to home maintenance, we pay special attention to certain areas of the bathroom. Caulk tends to crack and get moldy, and it needs to be replaced every year. After you shower, make sure the curtain or shower door is open to help air reach and dry it out.

Rain washes away more than just the accumulated dirt on the ground. If you suffer from seasonal allergies, or more specifically, allergies to mold, weeds, or grass, you may find that rainfall triggers your symptoms. Simply staying inside when it's wet won't get you away from these types of allergens, as they can come inside as well. So here's the thing: our noses can become very sensitive. "It only takes a few cells of pollen, mold, or an animal to trigger an allergic reaction," according to Michelle Huckins, M.D., assistant professor of otolaryngology at Rutgers New Jersey Medical School.

5.1. Indoor Allergen Reduction

You can also use a high-efficiency particulate arresting (HEPA) room air cleaner since the role of HEPA room air cleaner in reducing indoor allergen levels had been established in some studies. In the case of outdoor allergies, people can use air conditioning to keep the house cool without opening the window and avoid rainy days because the amount of pollen released into the air is diminishing. Therefore, staying indoors on days when the pollen count is high can give some benefits. Stepping further about strategies in reducing allergic symptoms, here in this subsection, we will provide practical aspects, especially alternation of indoor conditions by reducing indoor allergens. Suppression of indoor allergens minimizes allergic symptoms particularly among sensitive individuals. As mentioned previously, several strategies can ameliorate the possibility of exposure to allergens; indirectly reduce allergic responses in individual cases.

This can be done by keeping your homes clean and it is best not to have carpets, as dust and mites are easily trapped in it. However, if this is very difficult, it is best to vacuum carpets using an HEPA filter vacuum cleaner and do not forget to sweep in the hidden places such as under the bed and behind furniture. In addition to cleaning the house, allergens carried by rain are also contained in the air, so use an effective filter on the air conditioner in the room and also for ventilation can be beneficial.

6. Research Studies and Findings on Rain and Allergies

One study from Charlotte, North Carolina, concluded that 67% of 55 children between the ages of 11 and 18 experienced allergies during thunderstorms, compared to the same children on non-thunderstorm days. A second study from Madrid, that thunderstorms released high concentrations of certain fungal spores into the air. When those affected by allergies in Madrid were also tested for sensitivity to the four fungi, the tests came back positive. In 2007, a study of adults in the Journal of Allergy and Clinical Immunology found that thunderstorms had the potential to send more than 40 allergens into the air. The air then pushed those allergens on the ground into the air again, leading to pollens being released into the air. However, the publication hedges its bets, noting it's "unknown" whether the increase in allergens during inclement weather is enough to "provoke symptoms."

A research study conducted on 244 children in Kuwait showed rainfall had 36% higher concentrations of allergens in the air, leading to a correlation between rain and allergic airway inflammation. The study, reported in 2012 at the American Thoracic Society International Conference, suggests that rain causes allergens like dust, pollen, plant fungi, and mite feces to form more spores, which breaks them into small pieces that are more easily inhaled. Rain washes these particles down into the ground or surfaces, which in turn causes them to re-evaporate back into the air as smaller, more easily inhaled particles. A drop in pressure in stormy weather may also prompt the biological release of plant spores and increase skin allergies. Meteorologists shared similar findings about rhinitis, nasal allergy, and asthmatic experiences on windy and rainy days in Christchurch. Hay fever sufferers might experience a buildup of mucous in their own biometric barometer, their sinuses. A small proportion are believed to suffer migraines as a result of the changes. Interchanges in weather fronts triggers the release of greater than normal levels of plant-based histamine in the human body, causing swelling in the nasal passages and extra mucous production, which in turn affects sinuses, creating typical symptoms of flu and aging. Past Australasian research by the National Institute of Water and Atmospheric Research shows that high pollen count is likely to exacerbate asthma in some people. During thunderstorms in Brisbane in 2014, when changes in air pressure and humidity can be felt in weather fronts, the Brisbane Allergy Clinic wisely anticipated an increase in demand. Although hay fever and asthma patients should notice less severe symptoms once the storm clears and asthma patients carry their preventer medication at all times, anyone experiencing rare symptoms such as chest pain, fainting, persistent heavy breathing between asthma attacks should seek medical attention. Diabetics should also note wet weather results in an increase in risk of low blood sugar reactions.

6.1. Case Studies

As hay fever is caused by aeroallergens, notably grass pollen, any factors that increase the pollen load and hence exposure will potentially lead to an increase in symptoms in people sensitive to aeroallergens. This recent research focuses on grass pollen because you can develop pharmaceutical products for ingestion to enable significant protection for the general population considering grass pollen allergies. Allergic disease is a group of conditions in which the immune system reacts to substances that are usually (but not in all subjects) harmless and in most people causes no symptoms. In people who have an allergic response, the immune system produces an antibody (IgE) to the allergen, and this is then detected on the surface of mast (tissue) cells. If the same allergen-antibody-IgE complex is encountered, then the mast cell releases chemicals (including histamine) which, in turn, cause disease symptoms (the "late-stage response"). Organ systems that can be affected by allergies include the respiratory system (allergic rhinitis/hay fever (AR), allergic asthma, and conjunctivitis), the skin (urticaria, eczema), and the digestive system.

A brief discussion on some actual precipitation events and their impact thereon might further illustrate the importance of rain-induced allergens in the case of perennially sensitive individuals. Such individuals may, when dry, experience a relatively low degree of symptoms due to sparse local pollen concentrations. Most of the data and evaluation methods provide a means of reporting grass pollen counts on a daily basis with some regional data. There now exists a small number of good quality data sources providing wide-area representation of grass pollen, in the range of a thousand kilometers, at a sub-daily time scale. This is a suitable range as grass pollen can be transported several hundreds of kilometers from the emission sources depending on the met conditions. Some recent episodes of convective rainfall are presented from our records of more than 20 years of data from Europe and Australia.

7. Future Directions in Rain-Related Allergy Research

The roles that location, a climatic element like pollen season length, and other pieces of the symptom-puzzle remain very understudied, and while residents of some areas of America report significant worsening of their allergies during rain, those in other areas do not; it is essential for allergy sufferers, non-allergic controls, and scientists to begin addressing these myriad issues. Indeed, continued exploration must always be necessary, as these experiments have great potential to continue to inform the future directions of research on this extremely understudied issue. This work, as a result, has the potential to provide a necessary framework for many controlled experiments, as well as to open new doors and existing data up to important scientific reevaluation.

7. Future directions in rain-related allergy research. Though many pertinent and exciting research endeavors are currently ongoing among institutions across the globe, many questions remain about the role rain plays in allergy exacerbation, especially among allergy sufferers. For example, researchers still need to better understand mechanisms of nasal hyper-responsiveness to allow for the development of the protocols necessary to more concretely study these effects in chamber and challenge studies. Eventually, biomarker work will be used to start untangling gene rain responses versus season rain responses, among other issues.

8. Conclusion and Key Takeaways

The Impact of Rain on Allergy Symptoms: Causes and Treatment

1. Introduction

Allergies that are caused by the same inhalant during the changing weather will be exacerbated. "During weather changes, people can experience a worsening of allergic rhinitis symptoms," explains Sandeep Gupta, MD, respiratory allergist at John Scott Health, The University of Queensland, and Mater Health, Australia. One of the factors that may increase the concentration of allergens in the air is a heavy rainfall event. The rain will trap and remove the increased allergens, but soon after the rain, allergy sufferers may experience a daring awakening due to the increase of less elevated allergens, the world's worst. In the early morning, air temperatures can aggravate allergic rhinitis.

- The rain does not cause allergic rhinitis. - But since a number of microscopic allergens are produced in the air, they are often seen at peak levels before and during a large rain event. - The amount of mold spores increases significantly in the moist environment triggered by the rain. Mold spores are normally present in the atmosphere.

Causes of rainfall allergies

People have different allergic reactions. Some people experience sneezing, itching eyes, and coughing for a few days. Others have severe and more persistent symptoms. Some people only experience symptoms during specific times of the year, while others have symptoms all season long. If your body is sensitive to trigger environments, extreme weather and natural changes during the different seasons can worsen your allergic rhinitis or hay fever condition, particularly in the rainy season. This essay discusses the causes of allergic reactions and offers treatment for them.

The impact of rain on allergy symptoms

1.1. Overview of Allergies and Symptoms

Inside each person, the immune system mounts a robust defense from offending allergens that penetrate the nose or mouth and ultimately trigger inflammation in the mucous membranes causing swelling (and thus a stuffy nose), narrowing of the airways in the lungs (which leads to wheezing) and other symptoms. The branch-like immune cells that react to allergens are called mast cells, which release a mixture of chemicals, including histamines. It is these histamines that cause many of the symptoms associated with allergies. Some studies suggest that different weather conditions can affect allergy severity, especially if an individual happens to be allergic to outdoor allergens. Many people with pollen, mold, and dust mite allergies often find their symptoms worse in the rain. Rain showers not only shake loose copious amounts of tree, weed, and grass pollen from their parent plants, which then spread throughout the air and sneak into unsuspecting nasal and lung passages, but they also bring out higher levels of allergenic molds. In addition, rainfall can break down larger pollen grains into smaller, more easily respirable pieces, essentially bursting the original allergen into many more allergy-provoking little bits.

An allergy is a physiological response to an environmental substance—such as an outdoor weed, mold, or animal dander—that your body finds offensive and, in turn, forms an immune response aimed at defending it against these allergens. Common allergy symptoms can affect different systems of the body. Hay fever, for example, primarily involves the mucous membranes of the mouth, eyes, nose, and throat and can cause watery, itchy eyes; sneezing; and a runny nose. Allergies that target the lungs can cause asthma symptoms including coughing, wheezing, and shortness of breath. In some rarer cases, allergies can cause diarrhea and other gastrointestinal symptoms, as well as widespread hives. When your immune system senses an offending allergen, it triggers a cascade of symptoms.

2. Effects of Rain on Allergies

The effects of rain on allergies are two-track, in that what impacts an individual with pollen allergies may not necessarily impact an individual with mold allergies and vice versa. However, while these two different biological reactions do not overlap, they work together to produce an enormous amount of allergy signals, which will always come in tow with the rain. Rainfall can affect pollen levels in different ways, depending on the specific nature of the weather in the area. For example, there can be a small increase or decrease in pollen during a light rainfall, due to the fact that "rain washes pollen out of the air" while "rain can also worsen allergies after drawing pollen into the environment." Heavy rain is seen as beneficial to people allergic to pollen, as it washes away pollen from the environment, effectively minimizing the amount of allergens that are in the air.

It is well-known that allergies are common and they occur when the immune system does not recognize a substance, so the result is a reaction in the body. However, outside of these basic facts, many individuals are unaware that being outside on a rainy day can wreak just as much havoc on the immune system as being outside on a sunny day. But how is it that something as gentle as rain can spur allergens to act out against the human body? It's important to acknowledge that there are several environmental factors that can potentially heighten allergy symptoms, from temperature to wind speed; however, it is rain that is one of the primary culprits, as it has the unique ability to make life equally miserable for individuals with intact immune systems.

2.1. Increased Pollen Levels

Hay fever can occur all year long, but there are usually more cases in fall and spring as trees, grass, and even flowers pollinate. Another small flowering plant can cause big allergies in some people. Ragweed grows from the Gulf Coast to Canada, so it's a big problem for a lot of people. About 23 million Americans are sensitive to ragweed pollen, which can travel hundreds of miles in the wind. Ragweed releases more pollen in the summer and early autumn, and those pollen levels increase when it's too windy to rain. Unusually warm weather can cause plants to pollinate out of season too, releasing even more allergic pollen into the air. Balliet said she's seeing a lot of patients seeking relief from fall allergy symptoms earlier than normal.

There is one particularly unpleasant time when rain comes into play in a way that many allergy sufferers notice shortly thereafter. Pollen levels are often higher after the rain, which can be bad news for those with hay fever or allergic rhinitis. Rain can clean the air of pollen until the raindrops become overloaded and can then burst into smaller pieces called aerosols or microniculei that can cause an even more powerful allergic response. This occurs seasonally and in wet, humid climates. "Rain can decrease the amount of pollen in the air, at least close to ground level, by washing it away. However, light and variable winds will allow the smaller and lighter allergens to drift to the ground. This can leave allergens at ground level rid of rain, with levels higher than those at head level immediately after the rain breaks."

2.2. Mold Growth and Spores

The EPA and ASDS conducted this study in 2010, which discovered that during the rainy season, the amount of mold in the exterior air in Phoenix increases, along with the correlation between higher outdoor mold counts and increased amplified arid changes. Each year, Dr. Travis Miller offers useful information on this seasonal allergy phenomenon. His observation is quite accurate, as our research suggests that during the rainy time, the number of outdoor mold spores increases. Rainwater is capable of splashing mold spores heavier than air up to 1.5 meters in height. It takes at least 1-2 days following a rainstorm, up to a week in some situations, for mold to begin growing and start releasing spores. In other words, 1-2 days after a rainstorm, most places in the world, particularly in the summer when temperatures rise, are not completely dry and can continue to host and deliver wetness to molds. Also, if you manually remove the visible water spots, there are also various indoor hidden crevices in houses that remain wet and ideal for mold to develop following a rainstorm. Additionally, weekends are typically rainy and, in many countries, the days with the most severe rain coincidentally occur. Let's take a closer look at how much actual data on the relationship between precipitation periods and mold spore counts can be documented by monitoring outdoor permanent spore traps in these comparative climates.

When it rains, it's pouring not only water, but moist air. And then, it stays. As we have learned, humidity and extreme temperatures affect our airways' behavior. Mold is an outdoor allergen from the beginning of spring to the middle of winter, depending on where you live. Certain types of mold are found in every state. Mold grows continuously outdoors, reminding us to pay attention to the humid seedbed created by rain. Usually, as soon as you leave the house, you are hit by a distinct smell. During a rainstorm, that enhances mold growth. As a part of their lifecycle, molds secrete spores. With the air currents and winds produced during a storm, those spores are released into the environment, increasing the amount of potential allergens in your local air. It can take from one day to several weeks for these spores to reach a neighboring area, depending on distance and current conditions. Just because it's not raining also doesn't mean that there won't be more mold around than when it is raining, as moisture that sticks around after the rain builds up bacterial infestations. Some ways in which you can control mold illness by avoiding it are by sealing openings and cracks in your home, using an air filter, spraying and wiping surfaces with a cleansing solution, using a dehumidifier, and making sure you have appropriate insulation around your house during renovations.

3. Factors Contributing to Worsening Allergy Symptoms

Some medical studies back this up. For instance, a group of 42 people with grass allergies was found to have more severe symptoms after a suppressed sneeze was induced on a rainy day compared with a dry day, signaling that the interaction between the two plays a role in symptom exacerbation. Results from a study on 1,834 people allergic to ragweed found that self-reported increased symptoms after both grass and ragweed pollen on rainy days were associated with slower ragweed and grass pollen descent from the atmosphere. Aerobiology research has shown that rain can strip mold spores from a spore source and that these particles can then become the source of even more spores, hence contributing to an increase in outdoor mold spore levels, potentially causing symptoms.

Allergies occur when a person's immune system mistakenly treats a substance (allergen) as a harmful pathogen, signals for the release of histamine and other mood-setting chemicals, and directs uncomfortable symptoms like itching, sneezing, congestion, hives, and asthma to appear. These symptoms tend to worsen on rainy days, so sufferers may be confined indoors where additional allergens, like dust mites and indoor mold, can cause symptoms to worsen. On top of that, because outdoor allergens can be lifted into the air by rain, the atmosphere can fill with even more allergic inflammation-triggering substances (like pollen) after a storm.

Consequently, many individuals wake up or experience allergy symptoms during rainy weather, especially spring.

3.1. Airborne Allergens

Accordingly, wet and heavy rainfall following the release of detectable levels of pollen (during heavy storms, pollen can reach great elevations prior to rainfall) usually lessen airborne pollen levels. After rain, cooler moist conditions generally do not facilitate pollen exposure. It is thus generally accepted that unless the onset of autumn precipitation is also accompanied by plainly cooler conditions, airborne pollen increases are usually not rate limiting for allergic sensitization. Therefore, as long as there are around synchronous peaks of pollen release and precipitation generally occurring during the flowering phase to help reduce their airborne presence.

Besides pollen, several other biological organisms and their metabolites can trigger allergy symptoms; some of these are very different from pollen production. Pollen of various sizes is produced in diverse types of stamen (male flowers) and disseminated for pollination of female flowers. Pollen of many plants is carried by the wind at various levels, ranging from the ground to a few hundred meters, depending on the height of the stamen, to the sympathetic stigma (pollinated part) of the female flowers within the same or a different type of plant.

A substantial quantity of individuals have allergic diseases that are connected to exposure to environmental allergens. The disseminated allergens are involved in aggravating allergy symptoms, including allergic diseases such as allergic rhinitis, conjunctivitis, and bronchial asthma. This has frequently been named pollen allergy.

3.1. Airborne Allergens

3.2. Indoor Allergens

Dust mites are small bugs that dwell in mattresses, pillows, and other comfortable household items. These critters flourish in an environment with a relative humidity of at least 70 percent, and rainy weather may drive indoor relative humidity levels higher if adequate moisture precautions aren't taken. House dust mites may be found in any house, regardless of cleanliness. Although cold and dry outdoor air may provide some alleviation of allergy symptoms, maintaining comfort during the winter with heating systems can actually force more dust mites indoors. Very cold outdoor air warmed in the home can raise the humidity to root levels, stimulating dust mite development, regardless of the season. Vacuuming and the use of air filters cannot completely eradicate dust mites from the home. Consequently, it is critical to ensure a cold outdoor temperature by using air conditioning, a dehumidifier, or a humidifier tailored to the time of the year, in order to keep relative humidity between 30-50%. Many people with allergies are allergic to more than one allergen. Additionally, allergens vary from region to region. Keep the use of cotton and wool fabric to a minimum throughout the sign. Consider wearing sunglasses or changing your clothes and taking a shower to wash allergens from your skin and hair. Changing bed linens once per week may just eradicate dust mites from your bed. Regularly vacuuming and cleaning surfaces are also required. Additionally, it is recommended to eliminate carpeting and use allergen-resistant covers on mattresses and pillows. Ensure that the room is well-ventilated either immediately after the shower or while cooking to remove pollutants and moisture. Furthermore, monitoring accumulated moisture in basements, bathrooms, and kitchens and cleaning the surfaces in those locations can lengthen the lives of the building and its inhabitants. Use of a ventilation fan while cooking or showering, in addition, is highly advised. Additionally, it is advisable to ensure an indoor relative humidity of between 30 and 50 percent by using a dehumidifier, changing humidity levels, heating condensation, or drying the air in any additional spaces containing heat exchange-equipped central cooling systems.

Dust Mites

Mold tends to grow wherever it finds dampness, and during or just after a heavy rain, try to fill your nostrils with the scent of either your front lawn or yard. If the air has a strong, earthy odor, there's almost certainly some mold about. In some extreme cases, strong rain can cause flooding within one's household. Furthermore, since mold can also grow on interior walls and then invade theirtem, it may be significantly more challenging to keep it under control. Even if you can't see mold lurking just behind the walls of your bedroom or living room, it may still trigger allergy symptoms.

Mold Growth

When the weather outside is rainy, many may suspect that their allergy symptoms will improve since mold and pollen have trouble traveling through the air. It may come as a surprise to many that indoor environments can actually become especially potent sources of allergens during or after rain. This can be due to heavy humidity, increased moisture, and other factors that make it easier for pollen, dust mites, and mold spores to thrive indoors.

4. Strategies to Manage Allergies During Rainy Weather

Long-term allergy care. Symptom control with antihistamines, decongestants, and other OTC drugs, and possibly allergy shots or medication, are all treatment possibilities. Medical care. Allergy shots, also known as subcutaneous immunotherapy, can reduce allergen reactions and have long-term benefits. A primary care physician, an allergist, or an immunologist will administer the allergy shots over time. Allergy symptoms will most likely be reduced before the season begins by receiving treatments for eight to ten weeks. Allergies are prevented. Take any preventative action aimed at preventing allergies. You can create dust mites by refraining from using wall-to-wall carpeting, using allergen-proof mattress protectors and pillow covers, and wearing well-fitted masks when working outdoors. Keep your windows shut to keep pollens outside.

Before the rainy season, be stationed on weather apps and television reports to keep yourself updated on accurate forecasts. Additionally, plan your daily wear in advance and anticipate rainfall to ensure your outfit selection is optimal. Following this, wear a raincoat and use an umbrella to avoid getting wet, particularly your head and face. Third, once you arrive at home, dry yourself with an absorbent towel to avoid seriously damp clothing. Prevent the spread of pollen and mold spores by drying outdoor clothing in your laundry room or another room where it doesn't come into contact with other items. Mold, dust mites, and fungi can grow on damp fabric. Use an air purifier indoors to keep allergens at bay.

4.1. Medications and Treatments

Over-the-counter and Prescription Antihistamines. Many patients will get relief from one of these medications for a few hours. Unfortunately, antihistamines can cause drowsiness. Some of the older prescription antihistamines not only cause drowsiness but also can cause difficulty concentrating, a dry mouth, and in some, a rapid heart rate. Sometimes a skin test to a panel of antihistamines can guide the doctor to select the most effective medication. This method is called Gastro-Intestinal Allergy Skin Testing. At night, nasal sprays could be used with an oral antihistamine to increase symptomatic relief while the patient is sleeping. Some of the over-the-counter and prescription antihistamines include Fexofenadine (Allegra), Cetirizine (Zyrtec), Loratadine (Claritin), Levocetirizine (Xyzal), Desloratadine (Clarinex), and hydroxyzine (Vistaril).

The following is a list of interventions that could help manage symptoms when rain worsens allergies:

Allergy symptoms worsened by rain, and that can be helped with medications and medical interventions, include sinus congestion, sneezing, itching, and runny nose; throat itching; ear congestion and/or itching; and asthma. Symptoms at any time of year that are severe, interfere with normal functioning including sleep, and do not respond to treatment warrant a medical evaluation.

There is a large and growing market of medications available to treat allergy symptoms. The wide variety of medications available for purchase with no prescription can be divided into two groups: those for treating active symptoms and those for preventing future symptoms. The medications available by prescription are also used for treating active symptoms and preventing future symptoms, but offer additional approaches to care, including, for example, nasal anticholinergic medications that help clear mucus and glucocorticosteroids which can reduce sinus inflammation.

In the case of anaphylactic allergies, these symptoms cannot be stopped. If you experience an anaphylactic reaction as a result of rain, look for remedies for your specific allergy symptoms. Staying indoors and limiting movement during the rains can shield against airborne allergens. If you must go outside, make sure your rain gear is effective. Keep umbrellas, raincoats, boots, and other waterproof clothing dry and clean. Ensure that all entryways are tightly sealed and that rain does not pour in. It is best if another family member or friend is able to handle wet gear (outside the building) or at least in an area where the impacts are less likely to cause allergic reactions (house entryway). A large-coverage outdoor shower will help you remove pollen from your body before coming into your house. Trapping wet outdoor runners and letting them dry will help to clean the dropped substances. Heading to a different shelter or area if you encounter a heavy rainfall or storm while outside will help. Since back-pollution causes more pollen and mold to grow in basements and floors, use a small entrance to your home as much as practicable.

Obviously, the best way to avoid getting wet is to use an umbrella, coat, and boots during the rain. In order to mitigate the impact of rain on allergic symptoms, the most effective approach is preventive measures rather than actual treatment. It is necessary to make more efforts to prevent rain from causing allergic symptoms, which cannot easily be stopped. There are several proactive actions that can be taken to prevent such allergies, including some home alterations, lifestyle adjustments, and an emphasis on diet. Towel, heat curing pad-poultice, and air purifiers (especially ones with HEPA or Nano-Plasma filters) can be used to alleviate or prevent allergies.